Raw Food Diet

The Most Effective and Proven Diet Guide and Cookbook to a Healthy Raw Food Diet! (raw food, raw food breakfast, raw food dinner, raw food lunch, ... paleo diet, health, recipes, vegetarian)

By:

Debra Schmitt

Published by Shepal Publishing
All Rights Reserved
Copyright 2016, New York

Table of Contents

Introduction

The idea of eating raw food is not a new one. In fact, of all the species on the planet, it is only *Homo Sapiens* that cook their food, and even then, we have only been doing so since we learned how to control fire about 500,000 years ago. When we gained the ability to control fire, we also gained the ability to improve our lives drastically. Fire gave us the ability to better protect ourselves, to extend the time in which we could be active, and most importantly, it allowed us to explore new areas where the climates were colder and more hostile than the tropics where we originally evolved.

However, the discovery of fire also helped to drastically change our diets and how we prepare our meals. This in turn had an effect on the flavor and nutrients that we gained from our food. Many people have attested to the fact that the raw food diet has helped them to overcome illness, stay healthier and happier, and some even say it saved their lives.

The raw food diet is a diet where ¾ if not ALL your food is ingested raw. This seems like it should be easy to do, however, it's simplicity is what makes this diet so difficult to implement. Additionally, you will need a transition period where you slowly work your way up to at least 75% raw food, as jumping straight into this diet may cause some undesirable side-effects. However, once you have adopted the practice of eating raw foods, you will begin to feel the benefits, and before you know it, you will be energetic, optimistic, and positively radiant.

Chapter 1:
The Raw Food Diet

The raw food diet may seem like a modern construct, but diets like it have been around for millennia, and can be traced back as far as humans have been evolving. In the beginning, humans had no choice in the matter as we did not know how to control fire and therefore did not know how to cook. However, even after we learned how to control fire, there are still many accounts of people eating largely uncooked meals.

For instance, two of the most famous ancient Greek figures, Hippocrates (the Father of Medicine) and Pythagoras (famed for his Mathematical theories) were reported to have a diet that consisted of mainly raw foods. In the 19th century, the founder of the Vegan movement, Sylvester Graham, was also reported to eat mainly raw food which he saw as having massive health benefits.

The twentieth century also has its fair share of famous individuals who swore by the raw food diet. In the 1930's, Dr. Weston Price, a prominent dentist, attributed many major dental issues to the ingestion of cooked food, particularly processed foods. The middle of the century saw two well-known health nutritionists, Viktoras Kulvinskas and Ann Wigmore, also laud the benefits of the diet. They founded the Hippocrates Institute together in an attempt to popularize the raw food diet, and educate people on the benefits of eating raw foods.

Their advocacy paid off, because by the 1980's the raw food diet was slowly entering the mainstream population. However, it would be over 20 years before it really became popular, especially when more people began to realize the health benefits that come with the raw food diet.

Just what IS the raw food diet?

The raw food diet is a diet where the food you eat is not cooked above 118°F or 48°C. It therefore consists mainly of fresh and dried fruit, vegetables, sprouted seeds, soaked and rolled grains, nut-based cheeses, nuts and seeds. These items may not sound very nutritious, however, they provide almost all the nutrients that most nutritional specialists will recommend for you to have a healthy, balanced diet. However, many people are intimidated by the diet from the get go because the planning and preparation of these ingredients is more time consuming than with other meals. Additionally, these ingredients tend to be more expensive than normal, processed convenience goods. Nevertheless, the benefits of the diet cannot be ignored.

Because this diet emphasizes the benefits of eating raw or living food so much, it is important that you understand what happens when you put your steak under the grill, in the oven, or on a searing skillet. Understanding exactly what happens to your food when you cook it will help you understand that you are not really giving up on anything, all you are changing is your diet.

Advantages and Disadvantages of cooking

When you cook your food, you are processing or breaking down your food using heat. The changes that occur due to heating are both physical and chemical, which begs the question; Why would we want to do this to the things that we would like to eat?

The first thing that most people say is safety, because cooking kills bacteria and other organisms that could cause illness. Common foods that cause food poisoning are animal products including seafood and dairy products. Because bacteria strive between 41°F and 140°F (5°C – 60°C), to kill them you need to cook the food at a higher temperature. However, you must keep in mind that food poisoning can also happen to those who have not washed their produce properly or those who buy improperly grown or harvested food, especially when it comes to fruits and vegetables.

Certain alterations in cooked food are favorable, such as the caramelization of onions and foods that are high in sugar. The change in color in some foods, especially animal products, is also thought of as being a desirable side effect of the heating process. The breakdown of starches into their component sugars is also thought to be a desirable effect on cooked food. One of the least known yet beneficial aspects of cooking is that it can create molecules that make certain antioxidants easier for the body to absorb. This is especially true for molecules such as lycopene, which is beneficial in the prevention of cancer.

However, there are very many disadvantages to cooking your food that many people do not know about. For instance, with many foods, especially fruits and vegetables, you lose the natural texture of the food thanks to the degradation of polysaccharides in the produce. Another disadvantage of cooking is that it tends to kill all the naturally enzymes in the food that you are cooking, making it harder for your body to digest the food. It is believed that your body cannot effectively digest food without some of these naturally occurring enzymes, meaning that a lot of the cooked food you eat, especially fruits and vegetables, do not supply you with all of the nutrients that they could provide. This means that cooked food may make you overwork your pancreas, which could lead to low enzyme levels in the body later in life, not to mention a host of other health issues.

There is also the belief that the body can only produce a limited amount of enzymes in its lifetime. By making your body create more enzymes to try and compensate for the naturally occurring enzymes, it means that you could be depleting reserves that you will need later on in life, therefore shortening your life span. Studies have shown that people over the age of 80 years old have approximately 33% of the enzymes that an 18-year-old has. This deficiency in enzymes could help promote fatigue, a weakened immune system, and could even help to cause cancer due to irregular cell division.

Despite the fact that the raw food diet and its relationship to enzymes is still up for debate in the scientific community, the studies that have been carried out so far contain some worrying information, and therefore should not be discounted without consideration. There are those scientists that believe that the enzymes in food do not necessarily aid in digestion, and that they are digested along with the rest of the food as it is processed in the gut. Whatever the case may be, it is undeniable that people's health improves drastically when fruits and vegetables are added to their diets.

Chapter 2:
Is the Raw Food Diet Nutritious?

This chapter must begin with a warning: EVERYONE IS DIFFERENT. Your diet is largely dependent on your health requirements, and these requirements are usually unique to the individual. Therefore, when you first begin a diet, you cannot really approach it with a 'one size fits all' mentality (because as we all know, one size RARELY fits all). In most cases, the best diet for you would be the one you are most comfortable and happy with. In this case, it could mean that as much as 25% of your food is cooked, or it could mean that absolutely none of your food is cooked. It all depends on you.

You should understand that like with all diets, this will not be the silver bullet that kills all your health problems. Just like any other diet, if not followed correctly, you could end up with a host of health issues. The best way to approach this diet is not to think of the restrictions that are entailed, rather, think of the world of possibility that has been placed at your feet, and explore that world to the best of your ability until you find what is right for you.

Protein in the raw food diet

One question that many people who indulge in the raw food diet is "What do you do for protein?" This is usually because many people are under the assumption that the only way to get protein is through animal products, which are not prominent in the raw food diet. However, if followed properly, the protein intake in the raw food diet could actually *exceed* the RDA (Recommended Daily Allowance). This is because most foods contain proteins, even if it is trace amounts. However, most plant proteins are incomplete proteins, (proteins that do not contain all 9 essential amino acids) therefore, a combination of vegetables is often needed to satisfy the body's hunger for proteins.

There was a time when it was thought that plant proteins would not be able to provide the nutrients that the body needed. However, that is slowly beginning to change, as many doctors are now arguing that they may be even *better* for us. This is mainly because animal proteins must be broken down, then reconstructed to suit the body's needs (because they are complete proteins) whereas incomplete proteins can skip the first step, making it easier for the body to make the proteins that will fit its needs. The research into this area is still in its infancy, but some studies have shown this to be true, while others have gone a step further and suggested that animal proteins may actually *increase* the body's need for protein thanks to the first step of the breakdown process.

When it comes to the raw food diet, the best foods to supply you with proteins are:

1. Fruits

Many fruits such as tomatoes, apricots, raisins, and prunes, contain proteins with 8 amino-acids, making them as close to complete as possible. Other fruits such as avocadoes, dates, cucumbers and most berries will also contain a high number of proteins, making them an important source of protein.

2. Vegetables

Your vegetables may be able to supply you with all the proteins you need every day, however, it is always good to mix them with other things such as fruits, nuts and seeds to ensure that you get all the essential amino acids necessary for your body to function. Vegetables that are rich in protein include broccoli, carrots, garlic, green peas, Brussels sprouts, corn, and mushrooms.

3. Green Leafy Vegetables

These are a fantastic way to add protein to your raw food diet without the added fat and calories that some of the other options listed here contain. You could make them into a salad, create smoothies, or even make them into delicious soups. Some of the best leafy vegetables to get include watercress, kale, spinach, and romaine lettuce.

4. Nuts and Seeds

Nuts and seeds are like royalty when it comes to proteins. They are absolutely packed with proteins, to the point where many people who are new to the raw food diet tend to binge on them to help cover the protein deficit they think they have. However, this is not such a good idea, as the fat and calories that are included in nuts and seeds could have an adverse effect on your health. Some of the best nuts and seeds to use for protein include sesame seeds, cashew nuts, flaxseeds, chia seeds, almonds, pumpkin seeds and sunflower seeds.

5. Protein powders

There are some people that will not touch protein powders as they feel they contradict the essence of the raw food diet. However, for those who are just starting out, these may be a good way for you to ensure you do not deny your body the proteins that it needs to function. When choosing a protein powder, try to ensure that it is made from raw-food-friendly ingredients such as Brazil nuts and hemp.

Minerals and their sources

Other than proteins, there are a host of other nutrients that people are afraid of missing out on when they begin the protein diet. For that reason, listed below are some of the minerals that have given people the greatest concern, and the foods that they can be found in.

1. Calcium

This mineral is essential for strong bones and teeth, and can be found in foods such as bok choy, almonds, sesame seeds, flaxseeds, kale, figs and broccoli.

2. Iron

This mineral is vital for the production of blood in the body, and should be consumed with foods that have vitamin c to aid in its absorption. Foods that contain iron include kelp, squash, broccoli, spinach, pine nuts, artichokes and seeds such as sunflower, sesame and pumpkin.

3. Magnesium

Magnesium is often lacking in processed foods, yet it is very important to bodily functions. You can find it in kale, artichokes, parsnips, almonds, cashews, potatoes, pumpkin seeds, bananas and spinach.

4. Zinc

Zinc is vital when it comes to producing enzymes and accelerating the healing process. It can be found in seeds such as chia and pumpkin, cashews, chard, pumpkin, bananas and figs.

5. Vitamin A

This vitamin is needed for good vision, healthy skin, and for a robust immune system. Foods that contain Vitamin A include carrots, chilies, leafy vegetables and squash.

6. Vitamin B

B vitamins are found in many raw food ingredients such as nuts, seeds, tomatoes and avocados. However, it is important to note that vitamin B12 is NOT present in plants, making it essential that you get supplements if you are going to undertake the raw food diet.

7. Vitamin C

Vitamin C is essential for development, and healthy blood vessels. It can be found in capsicum, chilies, kiwifruit, strawberries and citrus fruits.

8. Vitamin D

Raw food diets often lack this vital vitamin due to the fact that most of the best sources for it are animal proteins. However, you could get vitamin D from the sun by spending at least 15 minutes a day outside. You could also eat mushrooms to supplement your time in the sun.

9. Vitamin E

Vitamin E is essential in protecting against cancer, heart disease and damage to the eyes. Some of the best places to get vitamin E are almonds, sunflower seeds, avocados, papaya and broccoli

10. Vitamin K

This is one of the most essential vitamins as it helps the body to create blood clots. It can be found in broccoli, leafy greens, green onions and cabbage.

11. Fatty Acids

Fatty acids are necessary for your body, especially if you would like to maintain peak brain function. The best raw foods that you can get fatty acids from are flaxseed, leafy greens, walnuts, squash and broccoli.

What exactly can be eaten raw?

There are a multitude of fruits, vegetables, nuts and seeds that can be eaten raw. However, there are some that you should be careful of (or avoid completely) when they are eaten raw. A few examples are given below:

1. **Alfalfa Sprouts:** these are eaten raw all the time, but you should be careful as they contain toxins that can lead to serious illness if too many are ingested

2. **Apricot kernels:** these contain cyanide, so eat the flesh, ignore the kernel

3. **Buckwheat:** buckwheat can cause photosensitivity and be very toxic, so try to avoid ingesting it

4. **Cassava:** some cassava plants and flours from these plants can be toxic

5. **Cruciferous vegetables:** these should not be eaten raw regularly as they contain chemicals that can cause hypothyroid conditions. These vegetables include

cauliflower, kale, broccoli, arugula, cabbage and Brussels sprouts.

6. **Dairy:** unpasteurized dairy products are not recommended, even though there are those that think it would be a good idea to use them. This is because dairy can contain harmful bacteria that cause disease

7. **Eggs:** another food with its proponents, the reason eggs should not be eaten raw is because of the possibility of salmonella in the eggs, which can make you extremely sick and even cause death in the elderly, children, and those with compromised immune systems.

8. **Kidney beans:** these should never be eaten raw, as they could contain the chemical phytohaemagglutinin which is a toxin

9. **Meat:** raw meat can be the perfect breeding ground for parasites, bacteria and viruses

10. **Peas:** some types of peas can cause neurological issues if eaten raw

11. **Potatoes:** they contain hemagglutinins which can reduce the blood's oxygen carrying capacity

12. **Rhubarb:** the stalks may be safely eaten raw, but the leaves are poisonous and should never be eaten

13. **Vegetable greens:** these should be eaten in a reasonable manner as many of them contain oxalic acid which can promote the formation of kidney stones and inhibit the absorption of calcium and iron.

Chapter 3:
The Raw Food Pantry

Many people who would like to begin eating the raw food diet assume that all they are going to be eating is salads for the rest of their lives, but that is not the case. Though there are a number of salads you will enjoy, there are also things like vegan pastas, wraps and even desserts that you will be able to eat while on the raw food diet.

Regardless of the composition of your diet (75% raw to 100% raw foods) you should keep in mind that to do it successfully you are going to have to expand your horizons. This is not only to stave off boredom, but also to prevent nutritional deficiencies. Foods that you should have as a staple when on the raw food diet include:

- Carob Powder and raw cacao nibs

- Fresh and dried fruits (from a respected greengrocer)

- Fresh juices

- Nuts and seeds (this includes nut milk, flour and butter)

- Oils (extra-virgin olive oil, coconut oil and coconut butter)

- Herbs, spices (organic and air dried) and condiments

- Protein powder

- Raw miso, nama shoyu, kimchee and sauerkraut

- Raw sweeteners such as agave nectar, maple syrup, coconut nectar, and honey

- Sea vegetables and seaweed

- Dried legumes

- Sprouted seeds and grains

- Vegetables

- Whole grains

There are those who are on the raw food diet that also eat animal products, but you have to get these from a trusted source. Animal products that may be included are raw eggs, beef, fish, milk and raw-milk cheeses.

There are a number of foods that you will need to get rid of before you embark on this diet, especially if you have decided that you are going to eat a 100% raw food diet:

- **Alcohol and Caffeine** – These do not belong on most raw food diets and therefore should be avoided. There are some wines (especially red wines) that qualify as raw foods, but you are going to have to dig deep to find an alcohol that you can enjoy with your meal if you embark on the raw food diet.

- **Cooked foods** – It is the raw food diet for a reason....no cooked foods, including canned foods and some dried produce

- **Processed foods** – if it has any ingredients that you cannot place or pronounce, then forget about it. These include refined flours and sugars, as well as anything with additives and food dyes

- **Soy and Meat alternatives** – These are usually processed at temperatures that exceed 118°F (68°C) and therefore do not fit the criteria for the raw food diet. However, if you are not committed to 100% raw food, tofu would be good to have in the cooked portion of your diet as it goes well with many of the other ingredients in the raw food diet.

- **Sugar** – Sugars should be avoided at all costs, especially processed sugars. However, it is a personal choice if you would like to do this. You could include natural sweeteners such as honey, maple syrup, or agave nectar.

You are also going to need a number of tools to ensure that you make the most out of the raw food diet. Even though there are many meals you can make using just a knife and a chopping board, there is basic apparatus that you will need to make your life easier. This apparatus includes:

- **A blender** – this is for those that do not have a juicer or food processor. If you have an immersion blender it would be even better, especially for less intensive tasks.

- **Dehydrator** – having a dehydrator is necessary, especially if you would like to try out a wider variety of recipes. You do not have to get one right away if you do not have one, but it is definitely an investment you should make.

- **Food processor** – this machine is absolutely essential for this diet as it makes chopping, pureeing, and blending so much easier and more efficient.

- **Juicer** – if you would like to have some fresh juice with your meals or just as a drink, what better way to ensure its freshness than making it by yourself.

- **Mandoline** – this is used to make julienned vegetables, ribbons and batons. Though it is not that easy to use, it is one of the best tools you can have in your kitchen, especially when you learn how to use it

- **Thermometer** – ensuring that your food is the right temperature is important with this diet. Therefore, you need to have a thermometer, preferably a digital one that reads low temperatures, to ensure that your food stays within the right temperature range

Chapter 4:
Breakfast Recipes

Now that you know a little more about the raw food diet, we can now begin to explore a few recipes to introduce you to the raw food diet. This chapter focuses on what has been called the most important meal of the day, and you will not believe just how good these recipes are.

1. Berry Banana Crepes

When it comes to appearance, it is only color that separates these crepes from their flour-based counterparts. Though you can use almost any fruit as a filling, this recipe uses berries as they add a unique sweet yet tangy flavor to the meal.

Ingredients

For the Crepes:

5 Ripe Bananas, peeled and chopped

Lemon juice from 1 lemon

For the filling:

1 cup cashews, soaked in water for no less than 6 hours, drained

Flesh of 2 coconuts

2/3 tablespoon Agave Nectar

3 teaspoons Vanilla Extract

4 cups mixed berries

Directions

For the crepes:

1. Put the bananas and lemon juice in a blender and blend until smooth and watery

2. Pour the mixture into 6-inch circles on dehydrator sheets

3. Dehydrate for a minimum of 6 hours, at 115°F (46°C) until flexible

For the filling:

1. Put the ingredients EXCLUDING the berries in a blender and blend until smooth, then put the mixture in a small bowl in the refrigerator until it thickens

2. Put two crepes on a plate and put some of the creamy mixture in the center

3. Top the cream mixture with the berries and roll or fold the crepes over it

4. Serve immediately

2. Apple and Cinnamon Oatmeal

This is a recipe that can be made with countless different fruits and spices. You should experiment with some other fruits such as pineapples or pears.

Ingredients

2 cups almond milk

1 cup rolled oats

1/3 cup apple butter

6 teaspoons Agave Nectar

0.5 teaspoons diced almonds

1 tart apple, chopped

Directions

1. Stir the almond milk, oats, butter, nectar and cinnamon in a small bowl until thoroughly mixed

2. Cover the bowl and put in the refrigerator for the night

3. Cover with chopped almonds and apple in the morning

4. Serve immediately

3. Sweet Granola

Perhaps the best granola recipe ever, this will definitely get you off to a good start in the morning.

Ingredients

6 cups rolled oats

1.5 cups shredded coconut

1 cup each of the following: sunflower seeds, chopped almonds, raisins

0.5 cup each of the following: pumpkin seeds, hazelnuts, cranberries (dried if possible), honey and Extra-virgin olive oil

1 teaspoon cinnamon powder

0.5 teaspoons powdered nutmeg

Directions:

1. Put all the ingredients in a bowl, other than the honey and oil, and ensure they are evenly mixed together

2. Stir the honey and oil in a separate bowl until they are properly mixed

3. Pour the mixture into the oat blend, and use your hands to make sure everything is coated properly

4. Place the mixture on four dehydrator sheets and dehydrate for no less than 4 hours, or until very dry and brittle

5. Store the granola in the Refrigerator or freezer in airtight containers until you are ready to consume

4. Blackberry Lemon Curd

This is a fantastic little pie that you can eat for breakfast or as a desert.

Ingredients

1 cup cashews that have been soaked in water for at least 8 hours, drained

2/3 cup diced coconut flesh

Rind and juice from 3 lemons

3 fl. Oz water

2/3 cup Agave Nectar

4 cups blackberries

Salt (to taste)

Directions

1. Put the coconut, cashews, lemon juice and rind and water in a blender and blend on high for at least 3 minutes (until it is smooth and creamy)

2. Add the nectar and mix thoroughly

3. Add salt and pour the mixture into a container

4. Firmly close the container and put it in the refrigerator until you are ready to eat then serve the curd in bowls topped with blackberries

5. Revitalizing Energy Bars

If you find yourself too busy to cook a proper meal in the morning, then how about trying this recipe.

Ingredients

1 cup each of the following: Pitted Dates, Pecans, Pumpkin seeds

0.5 cups of the following: Dried Cranberries, Shredded coconut

1/3 cup chia seeds

1/3 cup powdered flaxseed

¼ cup cacao nibs

¼ cup hemp seeds

6 teaspoons melted coconut oil

Directions

1. Cover a 9 x 13-inch baking dish with wax paper

2. Place all the ingredients apart from the oil in a blender and blend until the ingredients stick together

3. Add the oil to taste if the mixture seems too dry

4. Put the mixture into the dish and put it in the refrigerator for 2 hours

5. Cut the bar into 16 pieces then store the bars in the refrigerator and consume as needed

6. Apple Sauce

This recipe tastes just like a whole apple. Do not skin the apples if you would like to get the most out of them, and also if you would like to add some texture to the sauce

Ingredients

Water as needed

2/3 cup pitted dates

8 apples, cored and roughly cut

0.25 cup lemon juice (the fresher the better)

1 teaspoon powdered cinnamon

0.25 teaspoon powdered nutmeg

Directions

1. Put the water and dates in a small bowl and soak for an hour, then drain, putting the water aside for later

2. Place the dates, apples, and about 1/3 cup of the water from step 1 in a blender and blend for 30 seconds

3. Add the lemon juice and spices and blend for at least 1 minute

4. Serve immediately

N.B. The sauce can be stored for up to 4 days in the refrigerator

7. Almond Bread

This is a fantastic recipe to enjoy with a cup of tea or a glass of almond milk

Ingredients

6 cups almond flour

1.5 cups dried cranberries

1 cup powdered flaxseed

1.5 cups coconut oil or Extra-virgin olive oil

1 teaspoon salt

Directions

1. Put the flour, cranberries and flaxseed in a bowl and mix thoroughly

2. Add the oil and salt and mix until a dough forms

3. Press the dough on a drying sheet until it is at least 0.25 inches thick

4. Cut the dough into 20 pieces

5. Put another drying sheet on the dough and flip it over

6. Remove the top sheet

7. Dehydrate for at least 7 hours at 105°F (41°C)

8. Rice pudding

This is another great recipe that can be eaten for breakfast or as a dessert.

Ingredients

1 cup cashews soaked in water for at least 10 hours, drained

2 cups Almond milk

6 teaspoons maple syrup

Seeds from one vanilla bean

3 teaspoons vanilla extract

1 teaspoon powdered cinnamon

Pinch of salt

1/3 cup white chia seeds

Directions

1. Put all the ingredients except the chia seeds in a food processor and blend until smooth

2. Pour the mixture into a bowl and introduce the chia seeds, stirring as you do so

3. Cover the bowl and place in the refrigerator for 4-10 hours

4. Serve immediately

Chapter 5:
Soups and Salads

These are great for both lunch and dinner, and they are perfect to serve to friends and family.

1. Avocado Soup

This soup's gentle green color is complemented by fresh chives and cilantro. Its creamy texture and unique flavor are sure to make this a favorite.

Ingredients

4 avocados, peeled and pitted

1 cucumber, skin intact

2 celery stalks

Juice from 2 limes

0.25 cups chopped cilantro (the fresher the better)

6 teaspoons powdered cumin

3 teaspoons crushed coriander

3 teaspoons tamari

1-pint water

Salt and ground black pepper to taste

Chopped chives and sour cream for garnish

Directions

1. Place all the ingredients other than the garnish, salt and pepper in a food processor and pulse until smooth

2. Add the salt and pepper to your liking

3. Put in 6 bowls, garnish and serve immediately

2. Refined Mushroom Soup

This soup takes advantage of the meaty flavor of shiitake mushrooms, ensuring that even the most die-hard meat lover will enjoy this flavorful dish.

Ingredients

6 cups dried Shiitake mushrooms

5 pints water

6 teaspoons Nama Shoyu

Salt and ground black pepper to taste

3 teaspoons diced chives

Directions

1. Soak the mushrooms in the water in the refrigerator for at least 8 hours

2. Drain the water from the mushrooms using a strainer, squeezing the mushrooms against the strainer as you do so

3. Add the Nama Shoyu to the water, stirring constantly as you do so

4. Add the salt and pepper to taste

5. Throw away the stems from the mushrooms, cut the caps, and add them to the broth

6. Top with the chives and serve immediately

3. Avocado and Capsicum Soup

The color of the Capsicum is complemented will by the avocado, making this not only an aesthetically pleasing meal, but a great tasting one as well

Ingredients

16 seeded Capsicum

2 mashed avocados

6 teaspoons maple syrup

0.5 teaspoon grated horseradish

Salt and pepper to taste

Fresh basil, chopped into chiffonade for garnish

Directions

1. Put the red peppers in a juicer and throw away the pulp

2. Put 6-7 cups of pepper juice in a bowl

3. Stir the avocado, syrup and horseradish into the juice, ensuring that they are mixed thoroughly

4. Add salt and pepper to taste

5. Place in the refrigerator until chilled (about half an hour) and garnish with the basil

6. Serve immediately

4. Carrot and Peanut soup

It may sound unorthodox, but you will be surprised at just how much you will enjoy this delicious soup.

Ingredients

8 cups fresh carrot juice

1 avocado, pitted and peeled

1 sweet potato, peeled and chopped

½ jalapeño pepper, seeded and finely chopped

½ sweet onion, finely chopped

2/3 cup raw peanut butter

1 2/3 tablespoon Agave Nectar

Rind and Juice from 2 limes

1 teaspoon grated ginger

1 teaspoon crushed garlic

1 teaspoon powdered cumin

1 teaspoon powdered cinnamon

Mango chutney and 0.25 cups chopped cilantro for garnish

Directions

1. Put all the ingredients other than the garnishes into a blender and blend on medium-high until smooth

2. Place the soup in bowls and garnish with a teaspoon of mango chutney and some cilantro

5. Waldorf Salad

Named after the famous Waldorf Astoria hotel in New York City, this salad has been adapted specially to fit the needs of the raw food diet, and it tastes even better than the original.

Ingredients

2 apples, cored and chopped

13 oz. red seedless grapes, cut in half

4 celery stalks, chopped fine

1.5 cups pecans

3 teaspoons chopped mint (The fresher the better)

3 teaspoons maple syrup

0.5 teaspoon lemon juice

0.5 cup raw yoghurt

4 cups watercress (optional)

Directions

1. Place the apples, grapes, celery and pecans in a bowl and toss until uniformly mixed

2. Stir the mint, syrup, lemon juice and yoghurt in a bowl until uniformly mixed

3. Add the mint mixture to the salad and toss again to ensure a good, even coat and serve as is or on a bed of watercress

6. Kale and Broccoli Salad

This salad is both colorful and tasty, and is sure to leave your friends and family awestruck.

Ingredients

Salad Dressing

Juice and rind from one orange

3 teaspoons maple syrup

3 teaspoons balsamic vinegar

Salt and ground black pepper to taste

0.25 cup Extra-virgin olive oil

Salad

6 cups chopped kale

2 cups broccoli florets, roughly cut

2 cups cherry tomatoes, halved

2 scallions, cut thin

1 cup dried cranberries

0.25 cup pumpkin seeds for garnish

Directions

For the dressing

1. Add all the ingredients except the salt, pepper and the olive oil to a blender and blend until mixed

2. While you are blending, slowly add the olive oil until the dressing emulsifies

3. Add salt and pepper to taste

For the salad

1. Toss all the ingredients other than the garnish together in a bowl

2. Add the dressing and toss until it is coated evenly

3. Add the pumpkin seeds and serve immediately

7. Jicama salad with Cucumber dressing

This recipe calls for a rather unfamiliar vegetable, Jicama. A relative to the potato, it's ugly exterior hides a crisp, flavorful interior that will leave you wondering why you do not use it more often.

Ingredients

Dressing

0.5 cup almonds, soaked in water for 4 hours, drained

1 cucumber, peeled and chopped

1 garlic clove

3 teaspoons Agave Nectar

Juice from a lime

1 teaspoon crushed coriander

½ teaspoon powdered cumin

Salt and ground black pepper to taste

The salad

4 cups Jicama, peeled and thinly sliced

4 cups cantaloupe, cubed

2 cups halved cherry tomatoes

1 cup pumpkin seeds

3 scallions, thinly sliced

Directions

The dressing

1. Put all the ingredients other than the salt ad pepper in a blender and blend for at least 1 minute, or until smooth

2. Add salt and pepper to taste

The salad

1. Put all the ingredients in a bowl and mix thoroughly

2. Add the dressing, ensuring that it has evenly coated the whole salad

3. Serve chilled

8. Spinach and Mango Salad

This is a great salad to try, especially if you are new to the Raw food diet. The dressing for this salad can be used for a range of others, as it is tasty yet not overpowering.

Ingredients

Dressing

6 teaspoons balsamic vinegar

3 teaspoons Agave Nectar

1 teaspoon thyme, chopped

0.25 cup Extra-virgin olive oil

Salt and ground black pepper to taste

Salad

4 cups baby spinach

2 cups Arugula

2 Mangoes, peeled and sliced

2 cucumbers, diced with the skins intact

0.5 cups pistachios, diced

Directions

For the dressing

1. Mix the vinegar, nectar and thyme thoroughly in a small bowl

2. Add the olive oil slowly, whipping until emulsified

3. Add salt and pepper to taste

For the salad

1. Place all the ingredients in a bowl, except the pistachios, and mix thoroughly

2. Add the dressing and mix until salad is finely coated

3. Top with the pistachios and serve immediately

Chapter 6:
Entrées and Desserts

There is nothing better than a good entrée, other than a good dessert. These elements help to complement the perfect meal, and with the raw food diet, they help to add both nutritious value and an interesting intro and outro to any meal.

1. Coconut Pad Thai

Pad Thai has become one of the most popular dishes in the recent past. This version does not use noodles for obvious reasons, but still manages to capture the flavor and the texture of the original meal.

Ingredients

Sauce

9 teaspoons peanut butter

6 teaspoons maple syrup

6 teaspoons Nama Shoyu

6 teaspoons crushed garlic

3 teaspoons Extra-Virgin Olive Oil

1 teaspoon crushed chili peppers

Pinch of salt

Vegetables

2 cups chopped Nappa Cabbage

2 cups julienned coconut

2 cups finely chopped carrot

1 cup julienned zucchini

0.5 sweet onion, diced thinly

2 scallions, diced

1 chili pepper, diced

0.5 cup cilantro, roughly cut

9 teaspoons diced peanuts

Directions

For the sauce

1. Blend all the ingredients using a hand-held blender for at least 30 seconds

For the vegetables

1. Place all the ingredients in a large bowl (other than the cilantro and peanuts) and mix thoroughly

2. Add the sauce and mix, ensuring that the vegetables are coated well

3. Serve with the cilantro and peanuts

2. Vegetable curry with Nut Rice

This may be a time-consuming recipe, but you will have no regrets when the flavor explodes in your mouth. It is especially useful on days when you are hosting those that do not follow the raw food diet.

Ingredients

Vegetables

2 1/2 cups peeled and chopped aubergine

2 cups chopped Portobello mushrooms

1 cup broccoli florets

1 cup fresh peas

8 tomatoes, diced small

6 teaspoons curry powder

6 teaspoons Tamari

6 teaspoons olive oil

6 teaspoons fresh lemon juice

1 teaspoon salt

Curry Sauce

1 capsicum, seeded and diced

0.75 cup grated coconut flesh

0.5 cup shredded cilantro

1/3 cup water

1 minced garlic clove

3 teaspoons curry powder

1 teaspoon powderd cumin

1 teaspoon fresh lemon juice

0.25 inch fresh ginger

Salt to taste

Nut rice

4 parsnips, cut into chunks

0.25 cup pine nuts

0.25 cup almonds

3 teaspoons Agave Nectar

2 teaspoons olive oil

2 teaspoons white miso

1 teaspoon lemon juice

Salt to taste

Directions

Vegetables

1. Place all the ingredients in a large bowl and mix thoroughly

2. Place the mixture on dehydrator sheets and dehydrate them for 3 hours at 105°F (41°C)

Curry Sauce

1. Blend all the ingredients in a processor for at least 2 minutes or until smooth

2. Modify the seasonings to your liking

3. Add to the dehydrated vegetables in a serving bowl and ensure they are coated evenly

Nut Rice

1. Put all the elements, other than the salt, in a blender and put on low power until the mixture resembles rice

2. Top with the curry and serve immediately

3. Chocolate Brownies

This is great as a dessert, though it would also do equally well on the breakfast table.

Ingredients

1 cup of almonds, soaked in water for 6 hours, drained

0.5 cup of cashews, soaked in water for 6 hours, drained

1.5 cups pitted dates

2/3 cocoa powder

Directions

1. Cover an 8x8 inch baking dish with wax paper

2. Mix all the ingredients in a blender until they look like cookie crumbs

3. Transfer the mixture to the dish squeeze it down

4. Put the dish in the freezer for at least 2 hours

5. Remove the pan, flip it onto a cutting board, remove the wax paper, and cut into 16 squares

6. Store the brownies in the freezer for future use

4. Maple and Walnut Icecream

This is definitely going to become a family favorite, and it is so easy to make you will not believe how much free time you will have.

Ingredients

6 cups walnuts, soaked in water for 10 hours, drained

1½ cups liquid kept from the walnuts

1½ cups maple syrup

Directions

1. Put the walnuts, liquid and syrup in a blender and blend on high power until smooth

2. Pour the mix through a strainer and put it in an icecream maker

3. Freeze according to the manufacturers instruction.

Conclusion

As mentioned earlier in this book, the raw food diet is not something that has existed for only the last 20 years, humans have been eating raw food for millions of years, and it is only right that we try (for the sake of our health) to go back to eating as much natural, organic, RAW food that we can.

The recipes within the pages of this book are just a few of my favorites, and you will be surprised just how easy they are to modify to fit your needs. The salad dressings could be used in other salads, while many of the salads can be modified by adding or removing certain elements.

Whatever you choose to do with your meals, just remember that the world of the raw food diet is your oyster, and you can experiment and do almost anything with your food other than cook it. As you can see from the recipes above, the raw food diet does not have to be boring, and you could soon be reaping the benefits of all that raw foods have to offer while simultaneously becoming a culinary genius.

www.ingramcontent.com/pod-product-compliance
Lightning Source LLC
Chambersburg PA
CBHW071138280526
45787CB00003B/1334